GW00715920

BLUE/GREEN ALGAE, SPIRULINA AND CHLORELLA

THE TONIFYING, NUTRITIVE, DETOXIFYING GREEN WONDERFOODS

Woodland Publishing Inc.
P.O. Box 160
Pleasant Grove, UT 84062

The information contained in this booklet is for educational purposes only. Please consult a professional health care physician.

TABLE OF CONTENTS

FUNCTIONS OF MICRO-ALGAE

WHAT EXACTLY IS BLUE/GREEN ALGAE?

There are more than 1500 species of Blue/Green Algae. For our purposes, we will concentrate on Spirulina in detail. Chlorella, which is technically only a green algae, will also be discussed in more general terms. Both algae have exhibited similar attributes. Blue/Green Algae are unique in that they have the characteristics of both bacteria and plants. They have the uncommon ability to photosynthesize the sun to create reactions with the chlorophyll they abundantly contain.

Blue/Green Algae have been scientifically tested, and research strongly suggests that in addition to being a superior source of nutrition, these micro-algae may have potent anti-cancer properties, protect the body's cellular system against free radical damage and successfully treat diseases of the liver.

Proponents of Blue/Green Algae point to its effectiveness in clearing the body of heavy metals such as cadmium, lead and mercury. It has also been used to treat patients who are withdrawing from cocaine. Apparently, the chemical constituents of Blue/Green Algae help to provide nutritional support and curb drug cravings.[1]

Blue/Green Algae that have been collected in Hawaii and the Palau Islands of Micronesia have been cultured to produce an extract which is being tested against cancerous cells and the HIV virus. The sulfo-lipid content of Blue/Green Algae has shown significant action against certain viruses. Finding a way of using these compounds to fight diseases like AIDS depends on engineering a more effective route of administration. Oral ingestion of Blue/Green Algae for people with AIDS was not effective.

As a natural food supplement, Blue/Green Algae contains a very impressive array of vitamins, minerals and amino acids. Blue/Green Algae is a natural wonder food with health-giving properties whose benefits are just beginning to be realized.

Spirulina is a type of Blue/Green Algae and Chlorella a type of green algae. Both are also known as micro-algae. They are aquatic plants which contain impressive stores of nutrients vital to maintaining the health of human beings. Because they are both so rich in chlorophyll, they can be used in applications which call for the therapeutic actions of chlorophyll. Both types of Blue/Green Algae offer excellent chlorophyll sources.

CHLOROPHYLL CONTENT OF SPIRULINA AND CHLORELLA

Spirulina is a rich source of chlorophyll, which is a green molecule common to plant life. The greater amount of chlorophyll, the greener the plant. Sunlight activates certain ions in chlorophyll which are released and subsequently stimulate a series of biochemical reactions that result in the production of proteins and vitamins.

Spirulina or Blue/Green Algae contains more chlorophyll than any other foods. In addition, the chlorophyll content of these mirco-algae can be more than doubled in certain growing conditions.

Chlorella contains even more chlorophyll than Spirulina, therefore, less of it is required to obtain some of the same medicinal effects.

PROPERTIES OF CHLOROPHYLL

- Inhibits the growth of bacteria in aerobic yeasts and fungal infections, wounds and in the digestive tract.
- Deodorizes and sanitizes the body, and is effective against bad breath and a toxic colon as well.
- Can help to decrease tooth decay and gum disease when used orally.

- Works as a natural anti-inflammatory in conditions such as arthritis, skin inflammations, sore throat, pancreatitis, gingivitis and stomach and intestinal irritation.
- Builds the blood and nutritionally supports the body, especially if in a weakened condition.
- Helps to stimulate the regeneration of tissue.
- Promotes friendly intestinal flora which helps to ensure proper elimination and disease resistance.
- Has the ability to enrich the blood and treat anemia. The molecular structure of chlorophyll is quite similar to hemoglobin (red blood cells). Chlorophyll is sometimes called the "blood of plant life."

SPIRULINA

(Algae pratensis)

COMMON NAMES: Blue/Green Algae, Chlorella (chlorella is actually another type of green micro-algae).

PLANT PARTS: Whole Plant

VITAMIN AND MINERAL CONTENT: Spirulina is rich in protein, chlorophyll and essential fatty acids. It is also high in vitamin A, and the B-vitamins. Spirulina contains a rich supply of iron, magnesium, and phosphorus. It also includes calcium, potassium, sodium, vitamin C and E, RNA and DNA nucleic acids, and phycocyanin (blue pigment). Spirulina is the highest plant source of beta-carotene, vitamin B12 and gamma linolenic acid (GLA). It contains more beta-carotene than carrot sources and 250% more vitamin B12 than liver. Spirulina is comprised of 65 to 70% of protein and provides all eight essential proteins. While beef is comprised of 18% protein, spirulina is at least 65% protein. In addition, 80% of the protein content of Spirulina is assimilated by the body as compared to 20% for beef. The calcium content of Spirulina is 26 times that of milk. A detailed breakdown of Spirulina's nutritive content follows.

ESSENTIAL AMINO ACIDS:

Isoleucine	4.13%
Leucine	5.80%
Lysine	4.00%
Methionine	2.27%
Phenylalanine	3.95%
Threonine	4.17%
Tryptophan	1.13%
Valine	6.00%

NON-ESSENTIAL AMINO ACIDS

Alanine	5.82%
Arginine	5.98%
Aspartic Acid	6.34%
Cystine	0.67%
Glutamic Acid	3.50%
Histidine	1.08%
Proline	2.97%
Serine	4.00%
Tyrosine	4.60%

MINERAL CONTENT OF SPIRULINA

Potassium	15,400 mg/kg
Sodium	15,400 mg/kg
Phosphorus	8,942 mg/kg
Magnesium	1,915 mg/kg
Calcium	1,315 mg/kg
Iron	580 mg/kg
Zinc	39 mg/kg
Manganese	25 mg/kg
Selenium	Trace

VITAMIN CONTENT OF SPIRULINA

Beta-Carotene	1700 mg/kg
Inositol	350 mg/kg
Vitamin E (Tocopherol)	190 mg/kg
Vitamin B3 (Niacin)	118 mg/kg
Vitamin B1 (Thiamine)	55 mg/kg
Vitamin B2 (Riboflavin)	40 mg/kg
Vitamin B5 (Pantothenic Acid)	11 mg/kg
Vitamin B6 (Pyridoxine)	3 mg/kg
Vitamin B12 (Cobalamin)	2 mg/kg
Folic Acid	.5 mg/kg

CHARACTER OF BLUE/GREEN ALGAE: Tonic, Nutritive, Purifier, Tonifier, Detoxifier.

BODY SYSTEMS TARGETED: Immune System, Liver, Kidneys, Blood, Digestive (intestinal flora), and Cardiovascular System.

FORMS: Spirulina as well as other Blue/Green Algae are available in capsules, tablets, powder, flakes, freeze-dried crystals and extracts. Powder forms can be mixed with moist foods or liquids. Using a blender to mix the powder is recommended. Add the powder to the liquid slowly or it may stick to the sides of the blender. Capsules and tablets are somewhat easier to take. Sometimes, Spirulina is combined with citrus granules. Chlorella is available in tablets or pre-measured packets.

STORAGE: Blue/Green Algae may be kept in storage without a vacuum pack or any special preservatives for years. Freeze dried varieties are recommended.

REGULATORY STATUS: The medical usage of any algae is not approved in the United States by the FDA. In Japan, however, algae like Spirulina are routinely prescribed by physicians who recognize their intrinsic and significant nutritional value. Quality control in avoiding contamination is vital.

RECOMMENDED USAGE: Blue/Green algae should be taken in large amounts when unusual physiological stressors are present. Athletes, pregnant or lactating women and people suffering from diabetes, liver disease, anemia, or malnutrition should increase their dosages. Follow label directions. Doses for children should be reduced. Usually, smaller amounts of Chlorella as compared to Spirulina are used to obtain similar results. Chlorella is normally available in tablets or pre-measured packets. Freeze dried Blue/Green Algae is highly recommended for its potency and shelf life. Different types of micro-algae can be combined with no detrimental side effects.

SAFETY: Because Blue/Green Algae usually grows among water that may appear to be stagnant or unclean, it has been, on occasion, associated with bacterial contamination. If it is purchased from a reliable source, Blue/Green Algae should be one of the most naturally sterile foods found in nature. Some people, who do not need to build their systems and take excess micro-algae such as Wild Blue/Green Algae can become lethargic and feel debilitated. This particular reaction is not a common one and seems to be based on need and dosage.

HISTORY: SPIRULINA

Spirulina is a one-celled form of Blue/Green Algae and like Bee pollen, is considered by some to be a miracle food. Recognized the world over as an extremely valuable micro-algae, Spirulina promises to become a buzz word of the 21st century. Some food science experts believe that spirulina may well be the nearly perfect food of the future. Recently, scientists have looked at spirulina as an immediate food source for populations who lack adequate nutrition. It has the capability of producing twenty times the amount of protein as that of soybeans on an equal amount of land area. Spirulina has an amazing ability to synthesize excellent quality food concentrates more efficiently than any other class of algae. It far surpasses the ability of any single grain, herb or plant in its extraordinarily high nutrient levels.

The name of Spirulina is derived from the Latin word for helix or spiral, which refers to the physical configuration of the microscopic organism. It thrives and multiplies in warm, alkaline fresh water sources. These primitive organisms were among the first life forms to inhabit our planet. Scientists believe that three and one-half billion years of life on earth is encoded in the RNA and DNA sequences of Spirulina.

Spirulina is a micro-algae which is an organism which exists somewhere between the plant and the animal kingdoms.

The ancient Aztecs of Mexico used Spirulina as a food staple. Cortez and Fray Toribo de Bonavente, during the course of their explorations of the region, recorded that these native people gathered a "blue mud" from Lake Texcoco and made a type of sun-dried chip from it.

In 1964, Jean Leonard, a Belgian botanist who travelled the Sahara Desert, found a group of locals called the Kanembu tribe heating dark green chip-like food objects over their millet dishes.[2] Today, Spirulina is often grown as a mono-culture in man-made ponds. In 1990, one Spirulina production plant sent shipments of the micro-algae to the victims of the nuclear disaster at Chernobyl.

Russian doctors have long advocated the use of Blue/Green Algae for radiation exposure. Russian studies concluded that Spirulina promoted the evacuation of radionucleotides without causing the side effects so typical of other drugs. Additionally, it stimulated T-cell production, which helped weakened victims to fight off secondary infections.

Recent research has concentrated on the sulfo-lipid content of Blue/Green Algae like Spirulina. These sulfo-lipid extracts have shown some promise as treatments for lethal viral diseases like AIDS. Today, the notion of "we are what we eat" has spawned renewed interest in the therapeutic value of a whole host of natural substances. "Green Foods" which include Spirulina and Chlorella are rich in dietary nutrients, readily assimilated and have immeasurable value for health conscious individuals.

It has not been until the last decade that Spirulina has re-emerged as a valuable nutrient. It is sold today in powder form or as freeze-dried crystals.

CHLORELLA: A BRIEF OVERVIEW

Chlorella is an ancient, single-celled green algae and has many of the same properties as Spirulina. It differs from Spirulina in that is contains a little less protein, a fraction of the beta-carotene and more than double the amount of nucleic acid and chlorophyll. Generally speaking, it is more expensive that Spirulina due to the added processing needed to make its tough outer cell walls digestible. Additionally, because it is so small, harvesting requires centrifuge-type processing, which further adds to production costs. Keep in mind that to obtain equal amounts of chlorophyll, one must buy more spirulina than chlorella.

Chlorella is one of the most widely consumed nutrients in Japan. Apparently, because the Japanese are exposed to high levels of radiation and pollution, Chlorella is used as a de-toxifier. The Japanese cultivated Chlorella during World War II as a practical way to feed millions of their people during times of food shortages.

Chlorella derives its name from "chlor" for green and "ella" for small. It does not have the blue color of Spirulina and is a true green algae, with an extremely high content of chlorophyll. Chlorella is the richest source of chlorophyll on earth. In 1890, M.W. Beijerninck, a microbiologist in Holland was the first to develop cultures of Chlorella *vulgaris*. Like Spirulina, Chlorella has the ability to detoxify pollutants and heavy metals.

Regarding its detoxification properties, David A. Steenblock, D.O. has stated:

"The detoxification capability of chlorella is due to its unique cell wall and the material associated with it. The cell walls of chlorella have been shown to have three layers, the thicker middle layer contains cellulose microfibrils.... Chlorella has the unique property of picking up toxic substances from the surrounding environment (even in your body) and holding on to them. Other studies have shown that chlorella cell walls absorb and hang on to uranium and lead."[3]

Chlorella can also boast of an impressive array of vitamins and minerals, including 19 amino acids. Studies have confirmed that Chlorella can stimulate the immune system by enhancing macrophages which kill bacteria, viruses and cancer cells. It also helps to regulate cholesterol levels and promote superior health.

Like Spirulina, Chlorella has been shown to exhibit impressive immune stimulation through promoting interferon production and stimulating the activity of killer-T cells. While Chlorella is similar to Spirulina in its applications, it is considered by some experts to be better for people suffering from nutrient deficiencies or compromised immunity. Chlorella has been used for Chronic Fatigue Syndrome, and fungal infections such as Candida *albicans*. Because it contains more fatty acids than Spirulina, it is an effective artery cleanser and has shown to be effective in reducing cholesterol and preventing atherosclerosis.

Unlike Spirulina, Chlorella does not contain the phycocyanin which is responsible for the blue color of some micro-algae like Spirulina. It also contains a higher percentage of fat than other micro-algae, therefore it may not be as useful in treating obesity.

FUNCTIONS OF MICRO-ALGAE

Both Spirulina and Chlorella have a number of therapeutic and nutritive functions. They are both excellent sources of chlorophyll and each emphazises different nutrients. They can be taken together without any side effects.

CHLOROPHYLL AND BLOOD BUILDING

Because Spirulina, Chlorella and other Blue/Green Algae contain plentiful supplies of chlorophyll, they can be considered blood-building foods. Some recent clinical investigations have suggested that some porphyrins which are the ringed structures found in heme and chlorophyll stimulate the synthesis of the protein portion of the hemoglobin molecule found in red blood cells. It is thought that certain portions of the chlorophyll molecule may actually stimulate the body's production of globin.

Animal studies found that small doses of chlorophyll given to anemic rabbits stimulated the synthesis of red blood cells. In these doses, it seemed to act as a natural stimulant to the bone marrow rather than interfering with the actual chemistry of red blood cell production.

Interestingly, many elements of plant "blood" or chlorophyll resemble human blood. Some scientists believe that this chemical similarity is based on the fact that the process of respiration in mammals and photosynthesis in plants are interdependent. The oxygen/carbon dioxide relationship of both processes are inversely linked.

WEIGHT CONTROL AND SPIRULINA

Spirulina can provide the body with all the nutrients it needs while acting as an appetite suppressant at the same time. Most overweight individuals have indulged in a lifestyle typified by overindulging in too many refined foods including: white sugar, white flour, junk foods, fatty foods and an excess of animal protein in the form of beef, pork or poultry.

The pure type of protein found in Spirulina is believed to satiate the body's need for protein, therefore animal sources are not craved as frequently. When food craving are controlled, one can assume that nutrition is complete and the risk of overeating the wrong things is minimized.

Spirulina, like Bee Pollen is considered a complete and whole food. The notion that eating balanced whole foods eliminates the need for excess consumption of meats, fats and carbohydrates is firmly entrenched in natural medicine.

Additionally, Spirulina has been found to help stabilize blood sugar levels. Anyone who suffers from hypoglycemia understands all too well the connection between blood sugar and appetite. Drastic fluctuations in blood glucose can stimulate abnormal hunger, resulting in an excess consumption of carbohydrates. Studies have shown that when blood sugar drops too low, food that is subsequently consumed is more easily converted to fat stores.

Because Chlorella has a much higher lipid content than Spirulina, it is generally not used for weight management.

METABOLISM BOOSTER: THE THYROXINE FACTOR

Thyroxine is normally produced in the thyroid gland and is intrinsically linked to metabolic rates. Body metabolism determines to a great extent whether we burn calories or store them. Clinical studies conducted in Russia have discovered that Spirulina contains some thyroxin factors which may explain why it promotes weight loss.[4]

CHOLESTEROL LEVELS AND SPIRULINA

Japanese studies have found that Spirulina reduced both total cholesterol and LDL levels in Japanese volunteers with high cholesterol counts. These subjects took seven 200 milligram tablets after each meal.[5] The mucopoly-saccahrides (MPs) found in the cell walls of Spirulina are complex sugars which can strengthen heart muscle and protect the cardiovascular system against artery destruction. These MPs also help to lower the risk of cholesterol build-up in blood vessels by lowering blood fats.[6]

THE DETOXIFYING PROPERTIES OF BLUE/GREEN ALGAE

Blue/Green Algae have the ability to aid in the detoxification of all organs, particularly the liver. The high chlorophyll content of these algae can actually wash drug deposits from the body, help purify the blood of harmful contaminants and counteract the effect of damaging acids.

Research conducted over the last several years has found that Blue/Green Algae can help to offset the very deleterious effects of x-rays, ultra-violet light, radiation, and a whole host of chemical toxins. These remarkable organisms can remove heavy metals such as lead, mercury and cadmium from the human body.

Chlorella is particularly effective in toxin removal. Its multilayered cell walls are responsible for much of the plant's immune-stimulating and detoxifying properties. It can help the body excrete poisons not only from the blood, but the intestinal tract as well. Substances such as pesticides, insecticides, hydrocarbons and various radioactive substances can be detoxified by Chlorella.

Chlorella has been used to detoxify people suffering from PCP (polychlorobiphenyl) exposure. Studies in Japan observed 30 patients who suffered for PCP poisoning and took daily doses of Chlorella for a one year period. There was subsequent improvement in almost all of these test subjects and they experienced less fatigue, better bowel movements and improved digestion during their therapy.[7]

Chlorella has been used in other cases of chemical poisoning and is accumulating some impressive credentials as a detoxifier.

"Beside PCP, another very harmful chlorinated hydrocarbon insecticide, chlordecone (kepone), has been shown to be removed more than twice as fast from the body when Chlorella is taken by mouth. Dr. Pre of the School of Medicine, West Virginia University, did a study in which chlorella speeded up the detoxification of this toxin, decreasing the half-life of the toxin from 40 to 19 days. The ingested algae passed through the gastro-intestinal tract unharmed, interrupted the enteric recirculation of the persistent insecticide, and subsequently eliminated the chlordecone with the feces...Another example of Chlorella's detoxification powers is a study in which a brewer's yeast culture was poisoned and killed by the addition of PCP, mercury, copper and cadmium. When Chlorella extract was added to these toxic substance, the brewer's yeast remained alive!"[8]

In order to survive the continual onslaught of toxins we are routinely exposed to, our livers must function efficiently. It is liver tissue which filters out poisons circulating in the blood. Consequently, our livers can become damaged if we absorb excess toxicity from either chemical pollutants, alcohol or drug consumption.

Chlorella has demonstrated its ability to protect the liver from toxic damage due to a substance called ethionine. Ethionine is a compound which promotes fatty infiltration of liver tissue. A fatty liver is a damaged liver and does not function effectively.

Because we live in terribly polluted environments, the ability of a natural substance to detoxify insecticides, pesticides and other potentially harmful chemicals is vital to our survival and health.

BOWEL TOXICITY AND THE POWER OF CHLOROPHYLL

Most of us do not eat enough fiber or drink enough pure water, moreover, we continually clog our bowels with refined sugars, flours and fats. Our constant need to artificially stimulate our colons in order to have regular bowel movements testifies to the sad fact that we suffer from poor colon health.

Blue/Green Algae contains more chlorophyll per gram than any other known plants. Both Spirulina and especially Chlorella contain impressive amounts of chlorophyll. While most of us remember the Cloret's ads which claimed that chlorophyll could deodorize our bad breath, few of us are aware of its ability to detoxify the bowel.

Apparently, chlorophyll acts to create an environment that is unfavorable for bacterial proliferation. Chlorella has the capability of absorbing poisons trapped in the intestinal tract and promotes peristalsis as well. Peristalsis is necessary for healthy, consistent bowel movements.

"The intestinal tract (especially the small intestines) is lined by patches of lymphocytes that are probably stimulated by the chlorella cell wall material to increase their ability to destroy invading microorganisms.... Chlorophyll and Chlorella thus would seem to function best in treating colons that are suffering from anaerobic bacterial overgrowth syndromes...Chlorella cell walls stimulate the intestine's linings, and if taken for a few months, will gradually strengthen the intestine, thus eliminating constipation...Chlorella also alters the bowel's content of bacteria by increasing the number of certain healthy bacteria."[9]

In essence, the chlorophyll content of Blue/Green Algae sanitizes the bowel, helping to destroy the bacteria that cause gas and disease. Chlorella is particularly good for this in that it contains the highest amount of chlorophyll of any of the Blue/Green Algae. In regards to intestinal gas, if you use Chlorella, you may find an initial increase in flatulence.

"The stimulating and detoxifying effect of Chlorella on the bowel produces an interesting result at times. Many people will release more gases than usual for three to seven days after beginning to use it. It is believed that the harmful intestinal bacteria are fermented and destroyed. After this initial adjustment period, the bowel functions better, and the gas problems disappear."[10]

In regards to constipation, Blue/Green Algae, like Chlorella stimulates the lining of the intestinal tract and if taken long term, will eventually eliminate constipation.

"It has been demonstrated by many clinical cases that the administration of Chlorella Algae is effective for the treatment of constipation. Y. Saito thought of applying the promotive effect of Chlorella on intestinal peristalsis to treat persistent abdominal gas."[11]

IMMUNE SYSTEM ENHANCER

The immune system provides the human body with protection by using a number of remarkable strategies to defend against various and sundry foreign invaders. Whenever the body perceives the presence of a foreign organism or substance, it is aggressively sought out, disabled, attacked or actually digested. Blue/Green Algae have been shown to affect immune defenses by stimulating a number of actions.

T-cells, which are a type of white blood cell or lymphocyte, are stimulated by algae like Chlorella and Spirulina. These defense cells are especially vital for their role in activating specific immunity or antibodies to target antagonists or substances called antigens. The more T-cell activity, the better the immune system functions. Diseases like AIDS are directly related to impaired T-cell function, which makes the body susceptible to a number of potentially fatal diseases.

Blue/Green Algae also accelerate the reproduction of macrophages which are the "killer cells" of the immune system. Macrophages respond to infectious invaders by surrounding the foreign material both in the blood and tissues and ingesting it. The chlorophyll found in Blue/Green Algae also boosts the rate at which these macrophages move and seems to increase their appetite as well.

People who take green food supplements claim that if they begin early enough, infections such as strep and influenza can be effectively warded off or at least minimized.

INTERFERON PRODUCTION AND CHLORELLA

Interferon is an extremely important factor in fighting off disease. Scientists have concluded that by stimulating interferon production, the body's natural defense system against infection and carcinogens is enhanced.

Chlorella extracts have been able to increase the circulation levels of interferon for a certain length of time. The polysaccharides which have been isolated from the cell walls of Chlorella were found to affect an increase in interferon production in mice which protected them against artificially induced influenza.[12]

Mice that were infected with estomegalovirus and lymphoma-YAC-I and treated with Chlorella extract also showed increased levels of interferon and natural killer cell production.

Spirulina is a Blue/Green Algae that is easily digestible and can help to protect the immune system. The GLA content of Spirulina has been linked to the action of prostaglandin PGE1 which is believed to play a significant role in immune function.

TISSUE REPAIR AND MICRO-ALGAE

Studies conducted in 1930 demonstrated that extracts from green plants could stimulate the growth of new skin tissue in serious wounds. In 1937, chlorophyll had been singled out as the active substance responsible for this action. Subsequent testing was done with hundreds of subjects who had various wounds and burns. A number of topical ointments were used to promote healing. The chlorophyll was the only substance that consistently showed significant results. It is believed that the anti-infectious property of chlorophyll facilitates faster healing. Radiation burns and ulcers also respond to chlorophyll.

The fact that the chemical structure of chlorophyll is almost identical to human blood may also play a role in its efficacy in promoting tissue repair.

HIV AND BLUE/GREEN ALGAE

In a press release in a 1989 edition of the *New York Times*, the National Cancer Institute revealed that a party of scientists had discovered that the sulfolipid compounds of a Blue/Green Algae exhibited activity against the AIDS virus. Unfortunately, ingesting these sulfolipids orally neutralized their therapeutic effect. Nevertheless, finding a method to formulate and administer these sulfolipids effectively is currently underway.

What these scientists found was that cellular extracts from cultured Blue/Green Algae protected human T-cells from infection with the AIDS virus. In laboratory tests, pure compounds derived from these algae also proved to have significant activity against the HIV virus. It is the sulfolipid content of Spirulina and other Blue/Green Algae which is believed to destroy certain viruses. These particular lipids are contained within the chloroplast membranes of the organisms.

WHAT MAKES SPIRULINA BLUE MAY FIGHT CANCER

The substance that gives Spirulina its blue/green color is called phycocyanin and in some laboratory studies increased the survival rate of mice with liver cancer. Spirulina has an abundant supply of phycocyanin, which is a biliprotein. Finding blue pigmentation in foods is uncommon. The blue color reflects the chemical astringency of the micro-algae. The tendency of an astringent to draw compounds together may be reflected in Spirolina's effect on brain cells. The phycocyanin content of the organism is believed to pull amino acids together to more efficiently produce neurotransmitters, which are necessary for mental function and emotional health.[13] Chlorella does not contain phycocyanin but has exhibited other anti-cancer properties.

CHLORELLA AND CANCER

Several animal studies have shown that Chlorella demonstrates anti-tumor activity. This action has been specifically observed against mammary tumors, leukemia, ascitic sarcoma and liver cancer. Tests were administered on a glycolipid sample of Chlorella and its immune-enhancing effects were confirmed. Immune stimulation resulted from the stimulation of interferon production, which was observed in laboratory mice infected with estomegalovirus. Scientists are just beginning to realize the profound effect that the immune system plays in fighting and destroying cancerous cells.

MICRO-ALGAE: THE FOUNTAIN OF YOUTH?

The unusually high stores of RNA and DNA also known as nucleic acids found in Spirulina have been known to cause cellular renewal and to reverse aging. As a wonder food from the sea, Blue/Green Algae is fascinating to say the least. Maynard, Murray M.D. in Energy Agriculture has written:

"Of special interest is the fact that the aging process does not appear to occur in the sea. The comparison between the cells of a huge adult whale and the cells taken from a newly born whale will show no evidence of the chemical changes observed when comparing cells of other adult and newly born mammals."

SPIRULINA AS A SUPERIOR NUTRITIVE SUPPLEMENT

In a dried stated, Spirulina contains the highest sources of protein, beta-carotene and nucleic acids of any animal or plant food. In addition, the growing conditions of micro-algae can be manipulated to make these organisms even more nutritious. For example, the mineral content of Spirulina can be altered toward the maximum value for human nutrition by adding minerals to the water in which the algae is cultivated.

In addition, frequently people who have immune systems which are compromised have trouble properly absorbing vital nutrients. Much of the protein content of Spirulina is easy to digest and absorb. The protein digestibility of Spirulina is rated at 85% as compared with 20% for beef. Much of Spirulina's protein is in the form of biliprotein, which has been predigested by the algae itself. Some of its carbohydrate content has already been metabolized into rhamnose and some remains as glycogen, which is crucial to supplying energy reserves after digestion.

There is no question that spirulina protein is superior to animal proteins which have been linked to so many modern diseases. Anyone who is malnourished or is in a weakened condition due to chronic diseases like liver disorders can greatly benefit from the protein found in Blue/Green Algae like Spirulina and Chlorella. In fact, supplying the body with protein from Spirulina can actually decrease one's craving for animal meats.[14]

"By eating only 10-15 grams daily of protein in this form, the body normally becomes satisfied and animal protein is craved less. In addition, the severe liver damage resulting from malnutrition, alcoholism, or the consumption of nutrient-destroying foods or drugs can be treated effectively by this type of nutrition. Spirulina also protects the kidneys and liver; builds and enriches the blood; cleanses the arteries; enhances intestinal flora; and inhibits the growth of fungi, bacteria and yeasts."[15]

Several laboratory experiments have proven that Spirulina is an excellent source of Vitamin A. The high beta-carotene content of the algae is readily absorbed creating higher levels in the plasma and liver of test animals than synthetic beta-carotene.[16]

Because more and more Americans are becoming increasingly health conscious, emerging scientific evidence supports the nutritional claims of micro-algae. Green foods will undoubtedly become the whole-food supplements of the 21st century.

SPECIFIC ACTIONS ASSOCIATED WITH BLUE/GREEN ALGAE

- Stimulates macrophages to destroy invading disease organisms and carcinogens.
- Potentiates the immune system with its anti-tumor, anti-viral and interferon inducing effects.
- Helps to sanitize the bowel by detoxifying the colon and promoting the growth of friendly bacteria.
- Promotes tissue repair in wounds and burns and has anti-infectious properties.
- Decreases cholesterol levels and helps to lower the risk of cardiovascular disease.
- Works as an anti-inflammatory, helping to reduce the inflammation characteristic of arthritis.
- Provides superior nutritional support as one of nature's whole foods for anyone who is weakened by disease, alcohol or drug abuse.
- Helps to balance RNA/DNA (nucleic acids).
- Curbs the appetite and helps to stimulate the metabolism.
- Works like an antioxidant in detoxifying the body of pollutants.

COMBINATIONS THAT ENHANCE BLUE/GREEN ALGAE

Blue/Green Algae acts as a perfect complement to antioxidants and blood purifying herbs such as Red Clover.

PRIMARY APPLICATIONS OF BLUE/GREEN ALGAE

- •BLOOD BUILDER
- •BLOOD PURIFIER
- •CATARACTS
- •CHRONIC DISEASES
- •CHRONIC FATIGUE
- •DIABETES
- •FOOD SUPPLEMENT
- •HEPATITIS
- •HYPOGLYCEMIA
- •GASTRITIS
- •GLAUCOMA
- •MALNUTRITION
- •OBESITY
- •TONIC
- •WEIGHT LOSS

SECONDARY APPLICATIONS OF BLUE/GREEN ALGAE

- •Allergies
- •Anemia
- •Appetite Suppressant
- •Arthritis
- •Blood Pressure Disorders
- •Diabetes
- •Energy
- •Goiter
- •Gout
- •Hypoglycemia
- •Skin Problems
- •Liver Disease
- •Poisoning (heavy metal)
- •Ulcers

ENDNOTES

[1]Paul Martin, "Facts About Blue Green Algae," *Let's Live* March 1990, 26.

[2]Laquerbe, Bernard, et.al., "Mineral Composition of Two Cyanophyceae, Spirulina Plantensis and Spirulina Geitleri," *C.R. Acad. Sci. Ser.* D. 270 1970, 2130-32.

[3]David A. Steenblock, D.O., "Chlorella and Detoxification," *Let's Live*, March, 1989, 28.

[4]T.A. Babaev, "Thyroxine-An Active Principle of Spirulina," *Uzb. Biol. Zh.*

[5]Debora Tkac. *The Doctor's Book of Home Remedies*. (New York: Bantam Books, 1991), 154.

[6]Paul Pitchford. *Healing With Whole Foods*, 192.

[7]Steenblock, 28.

[8]Ibid.

[9]Ibid., 31

[10]Ibid., 29.

[11]Ibid., 32.

[12]Daniel B. Mowrey, Ph.D., "Chlorella: A Jack-Of-All-Trades For Your Health," *Let's Live*, February, 1989, 80.

[13]Pitchford, 191.

[14]Ibid.

[15]Ibid.

[16]V.V. Annapurna, Y.G. Deosthale, and M.S. Bamji, "Spirulina as a Source of Vitamin A," *Plant-Foods-Human Nutrition*. 1991, April, 41 (2): 125-34.